HAPPY FEET LITTLE YOGIS

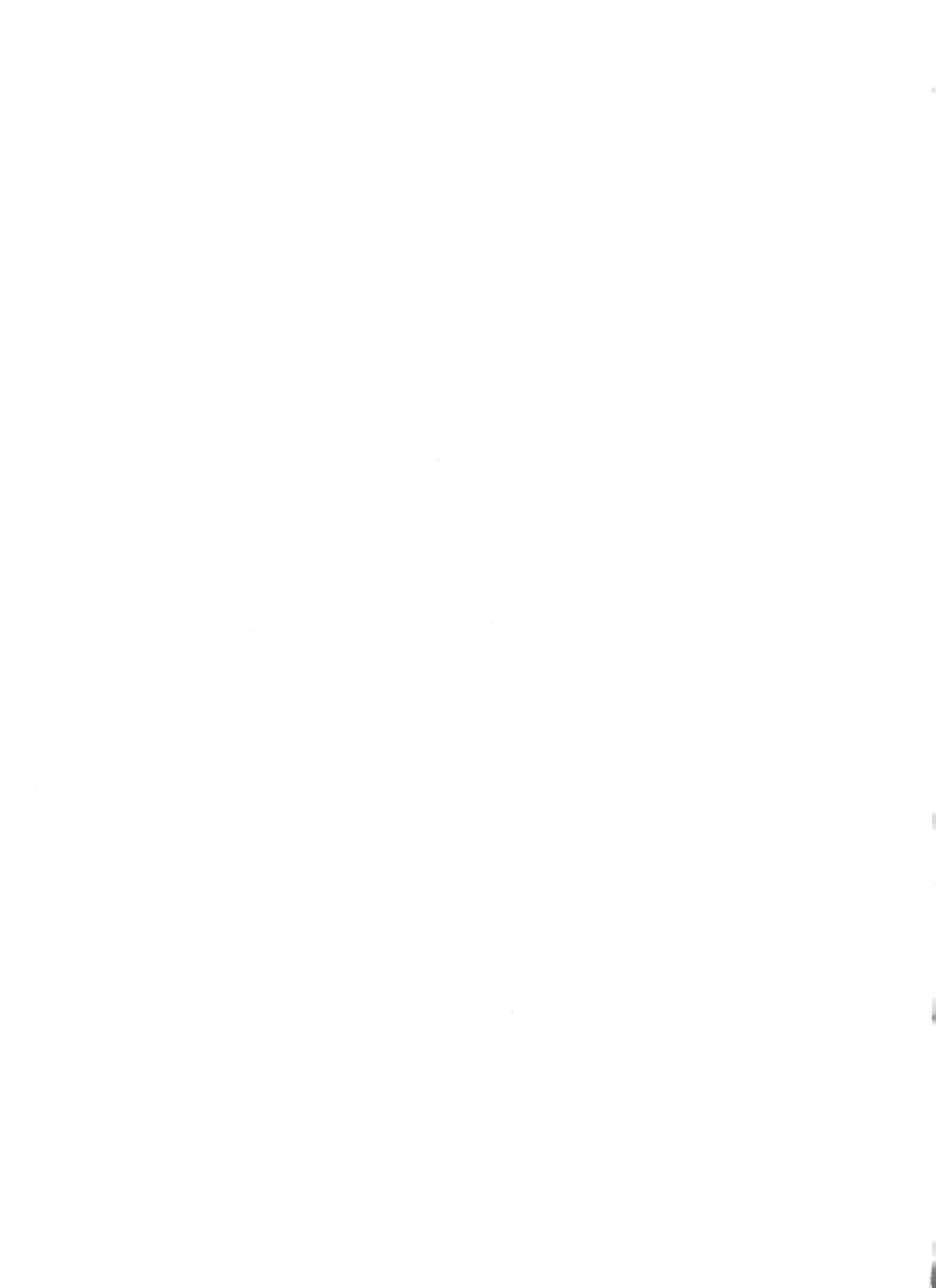

HAPPY FEET LITTLE 1 YOGIS

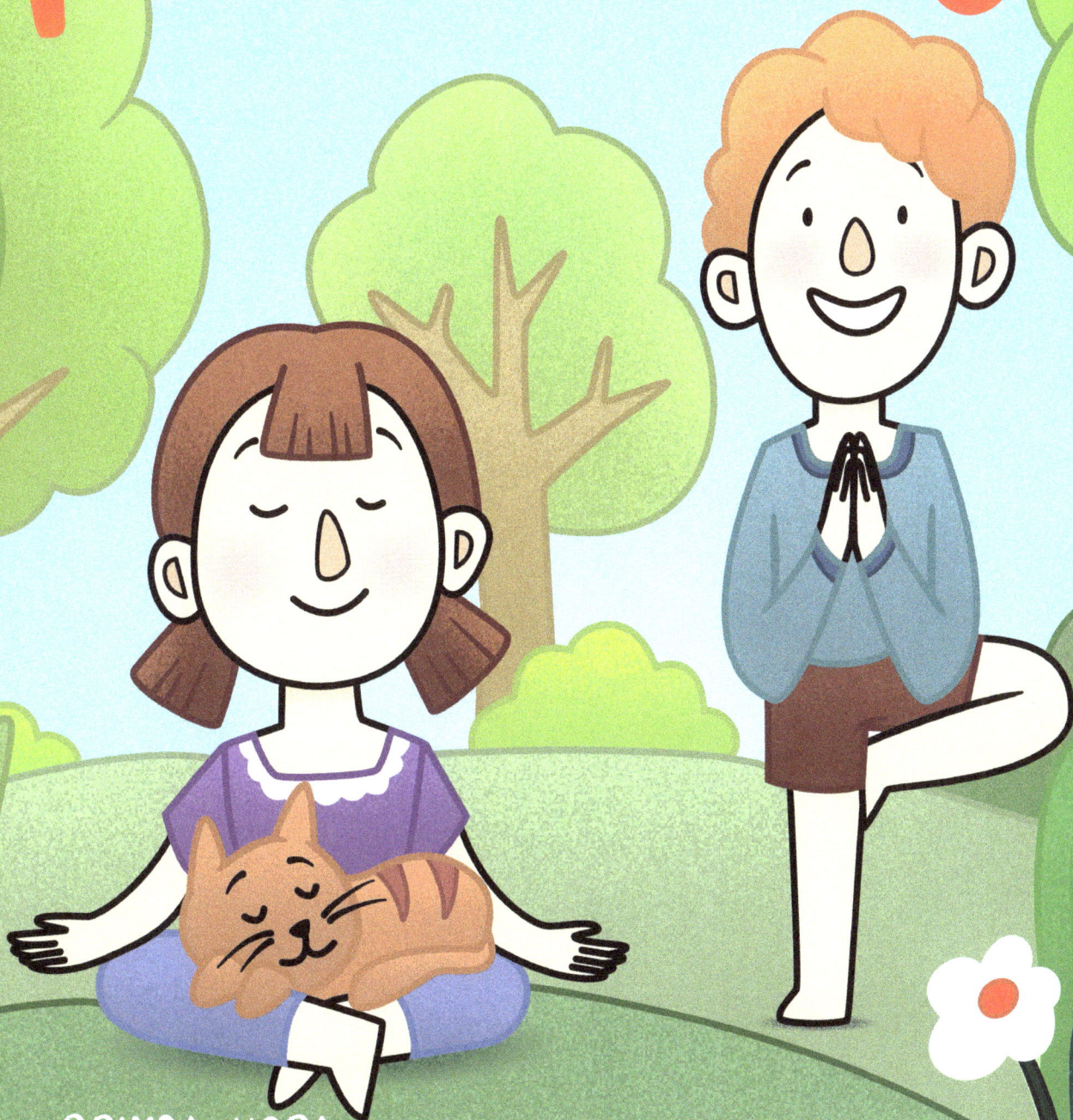

BRINDA HORA
AUTHOR

KATH JUNIO
ILLUSTRATOR

SEBB TURGO
DESIGNER

MOONSTONE

Published in Moonstone
by Rupa Publications India Pvt. Ltd 2025
7/16, Ansari Road, Daryaganj
New Delhi 110002

Sales centres:
Bengaluru Chennai
Hyderabad Jaipur Kathmandu
Kolkata Mumbai Prayagraj

P-ISBN: 978-93-7003-820-2

First impression 2025

10 9 8 7 6 5 4 3 2 1

Printed in India

WELCOME TO THE HAPPY FEET YOGI COMMUNITY!

We're thrilled to have you here, ready to stay HAPPY, thankful, and blessed! This special book is designed to bring joy to you and your loved ones. Filled with love and happiness, it's a unique activity book for children aged 3 years and above. As your little ones colour, they will practice motor control, develop critical thinking skills and explore yoga poses.

During the process of colouring and practising poses, they develop **critical thinking** by asking thoughtful questions like, *"How does this pose make me feel?"* or *"What does my body need in this moment?"* These questions help kids tune in to their bodies and start developing thoughtful reflection. The process of deciding how to colour each pose and imagining its benefits also strengthens their ability to think ahead, analyse actions, and make decisions—skills that will benefit them in many areas of life.

The book also encourages the development of **mind and motor skills**. Colouring builds focus and fine motor control, while yoga enhances balance, coordination, and body awareness. Together, these activities promote hand-eye coordination, muscle memory, and mindful movement.

Parents are encouraged to join in—guiding Little Yogis through poses, supporting their creativity, and making the experience fun and meaningful. Every child is a Yogi in their own way—a *Happy Feet 'Little' Yogi*.

These poses help children breathe, stretch, and strengthen while learning to tune into their bodies. For the best experience, practice yoga on a light tummy.

Ready to begin? Let's explore focus, mindfulness, and creativity—one breath, one pose, and one colour at a time!

SCAN TO WATCH
THE VIDEOS ONLINE

YOGI BREATH

Once upon a time, in a land of giggles and wiggles, there were
Happy Feet 'Little' Yogis like you! Ready for a special journey?

Find a cosy spot—on a soft mat, fluffy carpet, or smooth floor.
Cross your legs and get comfy.

Place one hand on your belly and the other on your heart.
Close your eyes and take a deep breath, feeling your belly
and heart rise. Can you sense the magic?

Let's say something wonderful together:

"I AM GROUNDED!"

This means we feel strong and calm.
Take a few more breaths,
then open your eyes. You did it!

You're a Little Yogi with a Happy Heart.
Ready to explore? Let's yoga!

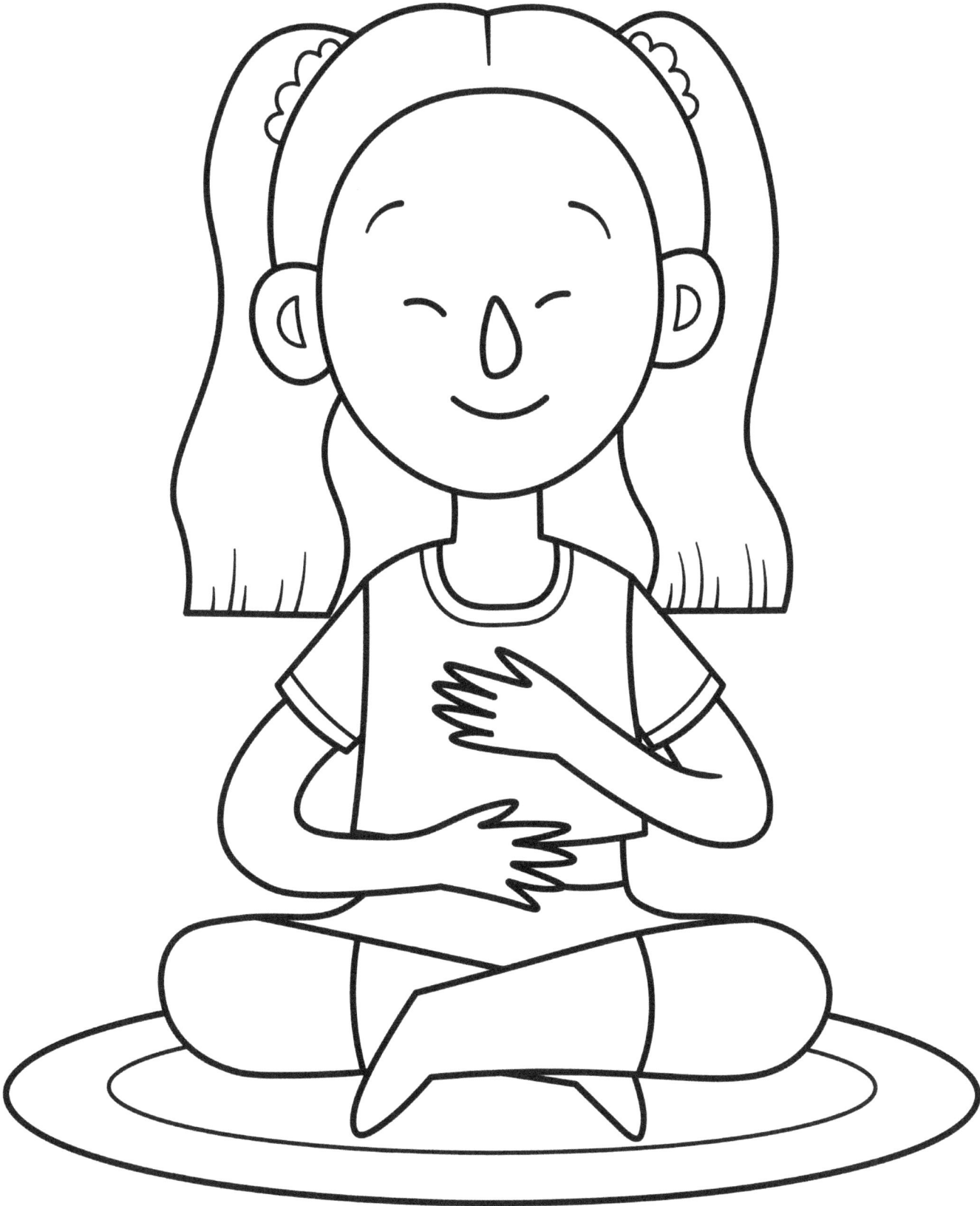

BALLOON BREATHING

Now that we're grounded, open your eyes and bring your
hands together in front of your chest, as if holding a balloon
ready to be filled with our breath.

Ready for a magical adventure? Take a big breath in through your nose,
and as you breathe out through your mouth, imagine your balloon growing
bigger. Inhale deeply, exhale, and see how big your balloon can get.
Continue for a few rounds.

When you're ready, let your balloon float away.
Wave your hands like a balloon soaring high. It's so much fun!

As you breathe, stay calm and relaxed. Let's say together:

"I AM AWARE!"

This means we're focusing on our breath and feelings.

Keep practising Happy Feet 'Little' Yogis.
Every breath is a new adventure!

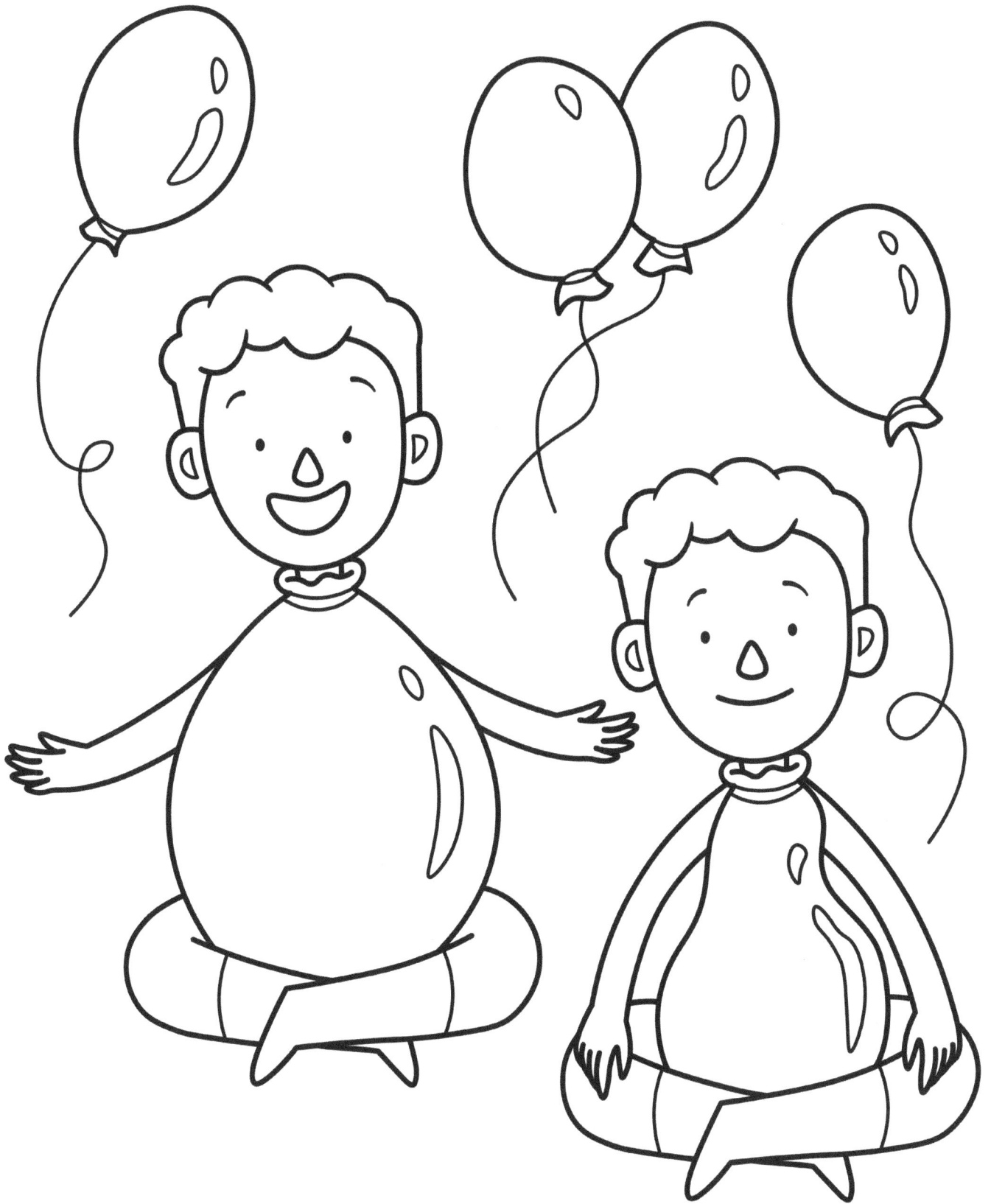

FINGER BREATHING

Alright, let's do one more fun breathing
exercise before our yoga poses. Ready?

Extend one hand in front of you, fingers stretched out like a mountain.
Use the index finger of your other hand to 'climb' up the mountain
as you breathe in through your nose. When you reach the top,
breathe out through your mouth and 'climb' back down.

Take your time and enjoy the climb. Feel your lungs expand
with each breath. Afterwards, relax and notice how you feel.

Let's say together:

"I AM CALM!"

Feel the calmness like sunshine on a quiet morning.

Great job, Happy Feet 'Little' Yogis!
Ready for our next yoga adventure? Let's go!

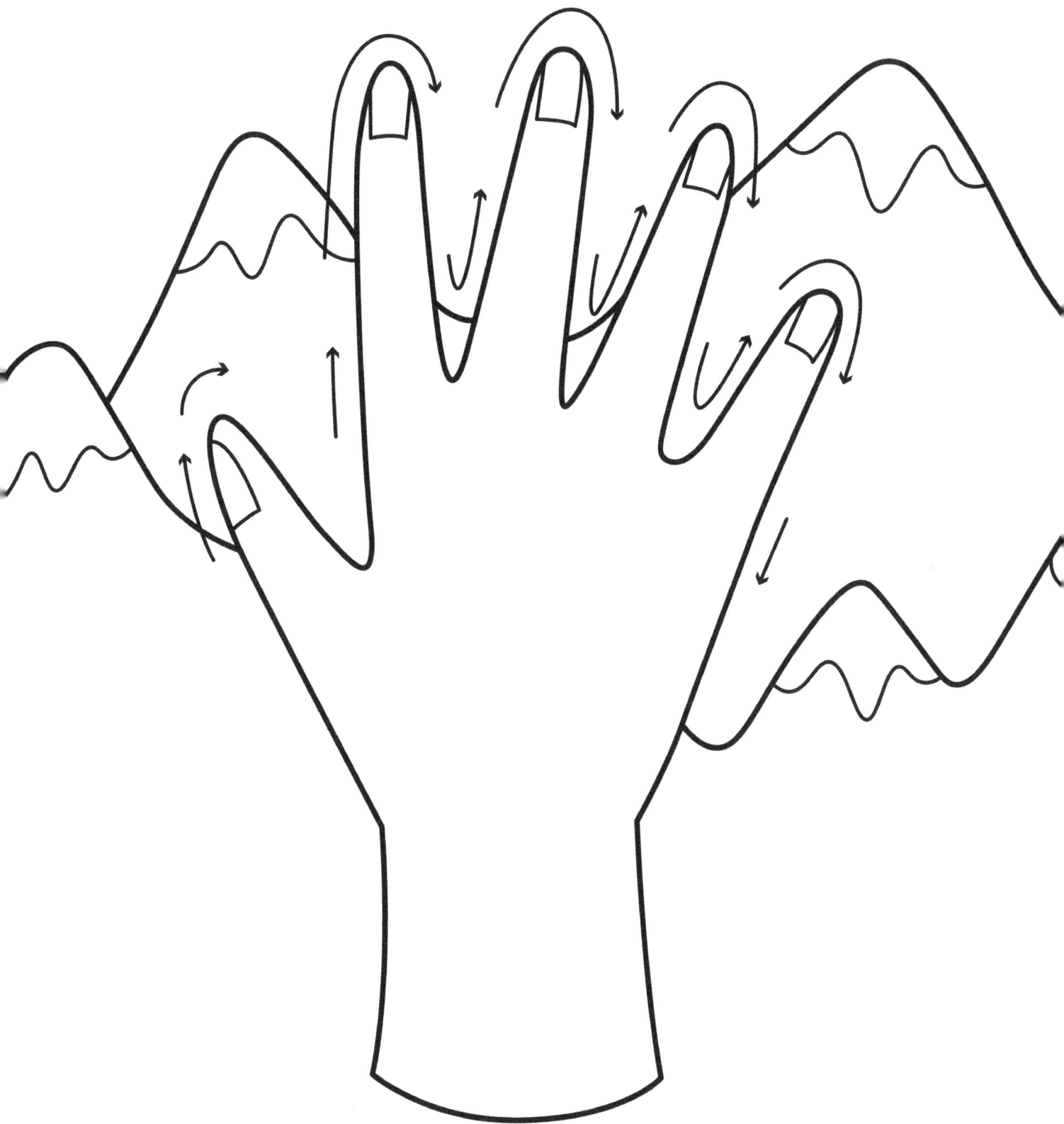

CHILD'S POSE

Happy Feet 'Little' Yogis, ready to stretch and feel amazing? Let's do it!

Find a comfy spot on your mat or the floor. Bend your knees and rest your hips on your heels. Spread your knees apart and extend your arms forward. Slowly lower your belly and chest towards the floor, keeping your arms straight.

Notice the stretch in your spine and the relaxation in your body. Stay in Child's Pose for at least 15 seconds or as long as you like. This pose increases blood flow to your hips, stretches your upper body and spine. It calms your mind and can even aid digestion!

Let's say an affirmation together:

"I AM WHERE I AM SUPPOSED TO BE!"

Feel the peace and comfort of being in the moment. Take a deep breath in and relax even more as you breathe out.

You're doing great, Little Yogis! When you're ready, come out of the pose and get ready for more exciting yoga adventures. Are you excited? Let's continue!

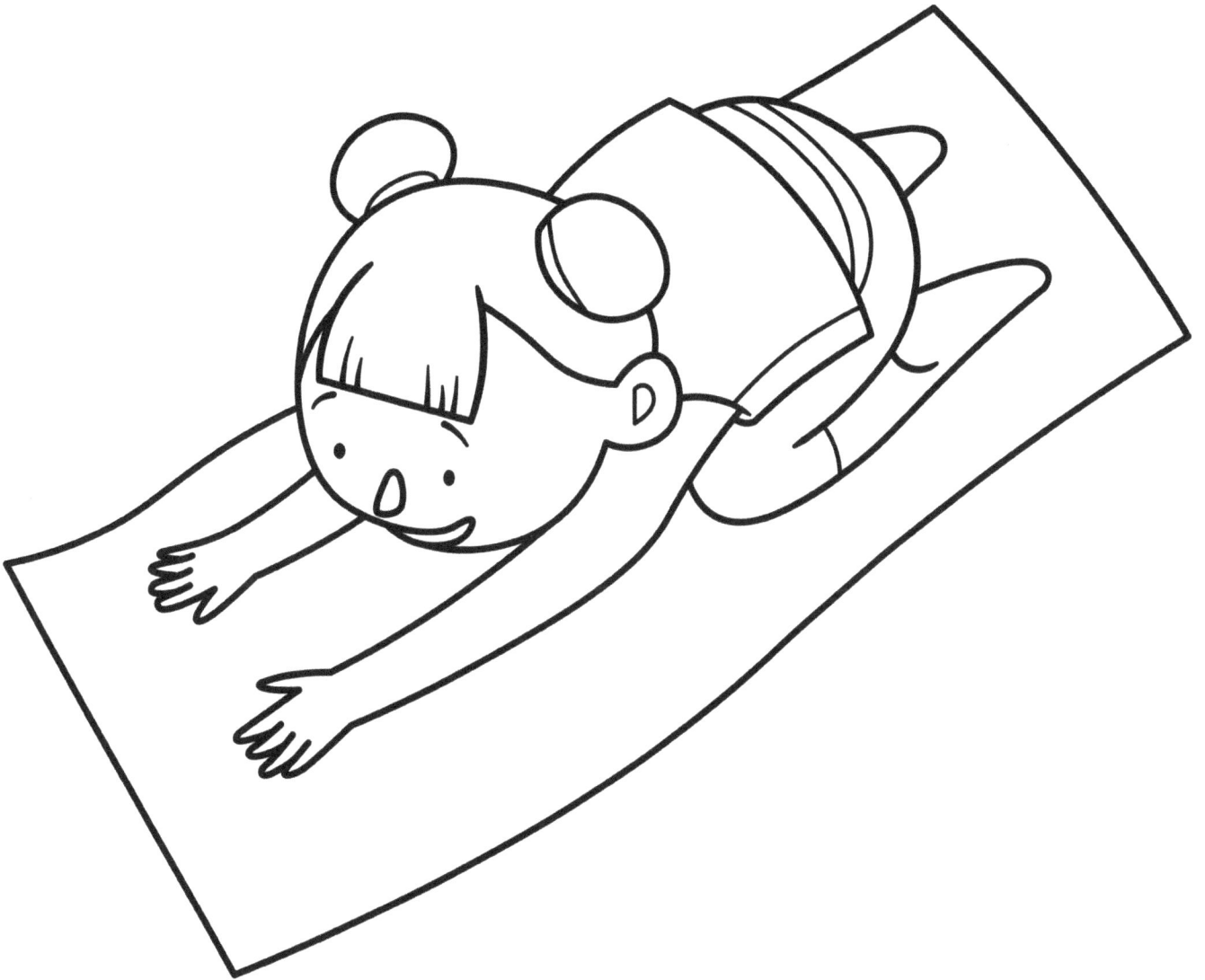

COW'S POSE

This sounds like so much fun doesn't it, Happy Feet 'Little' Yogis?
Ready to stretch and make some animal sounds? Let's go!

Sit on your mat or the floor with your knees bent and slightly apart.
Place your palms on the mat too, creating a "square" shape with your body
—two palms and two knees.

Take a deep breath in through your nose.
As you breathe in, arch your back and open your chest,
looking up. Can you make a big **MOOOOO** like a cow?
Let's hear it!

Let's say something wonderful together:

"I AM KIND!"

Feel the kindness spreading through you like sunshine.
Enjoy the exercise and get ready for the next pose.

Now, get ready to unleash your inner
cat in the next pose. **MEOOOW!!!**

Let's keep having fun and exploring yoga together!

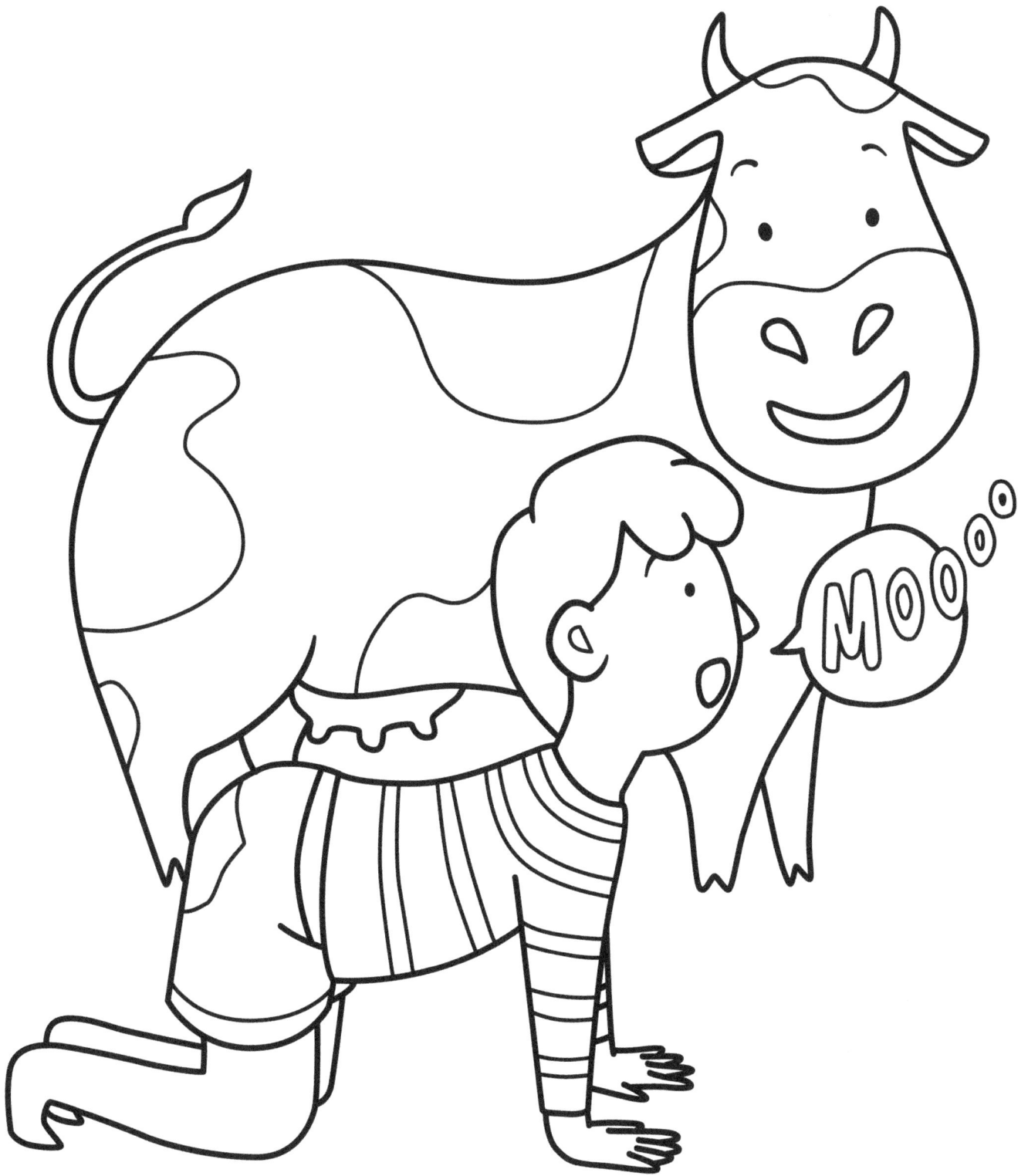

CAT'S POSE

You're doing brilliantly, Happy Feet 'Little' Yogis! Ready to continue
our fun yoga adventure with Cat Pose and Cow Pose? Let's go!

Start in the "on all fours" position—palms and knees
on the mat with a little space between them.

Cat Pose: Take a deep breath in. As you exhale,
round your back towards the sky, bring your chin to your chest,
and make a big **MEOOOWW** sound like a cat.
Feel the stretch in your spine and belly.

Cow Pose: Inhale deeply. As you breathe in,
arch your back, open your chest, and lift your head high,
making a big **MOOOOO** sound like a cow. Feel the stretch
in your spine going the other way.

Let's move like a Cat... now a Cow – nice and slow, we know how!
Stretch your back and tummy too, they are getting strong and you stand tall,
like the bravest of them all.

Once done, let's say together:

"I AM DOING MY BEST!"

Feel proud of yourself for trying new poses and giving your best.

Keep practising and having fun, Happy Feet 'Little' Yogis!
Let's continue our yoga journey with happiness and joy!

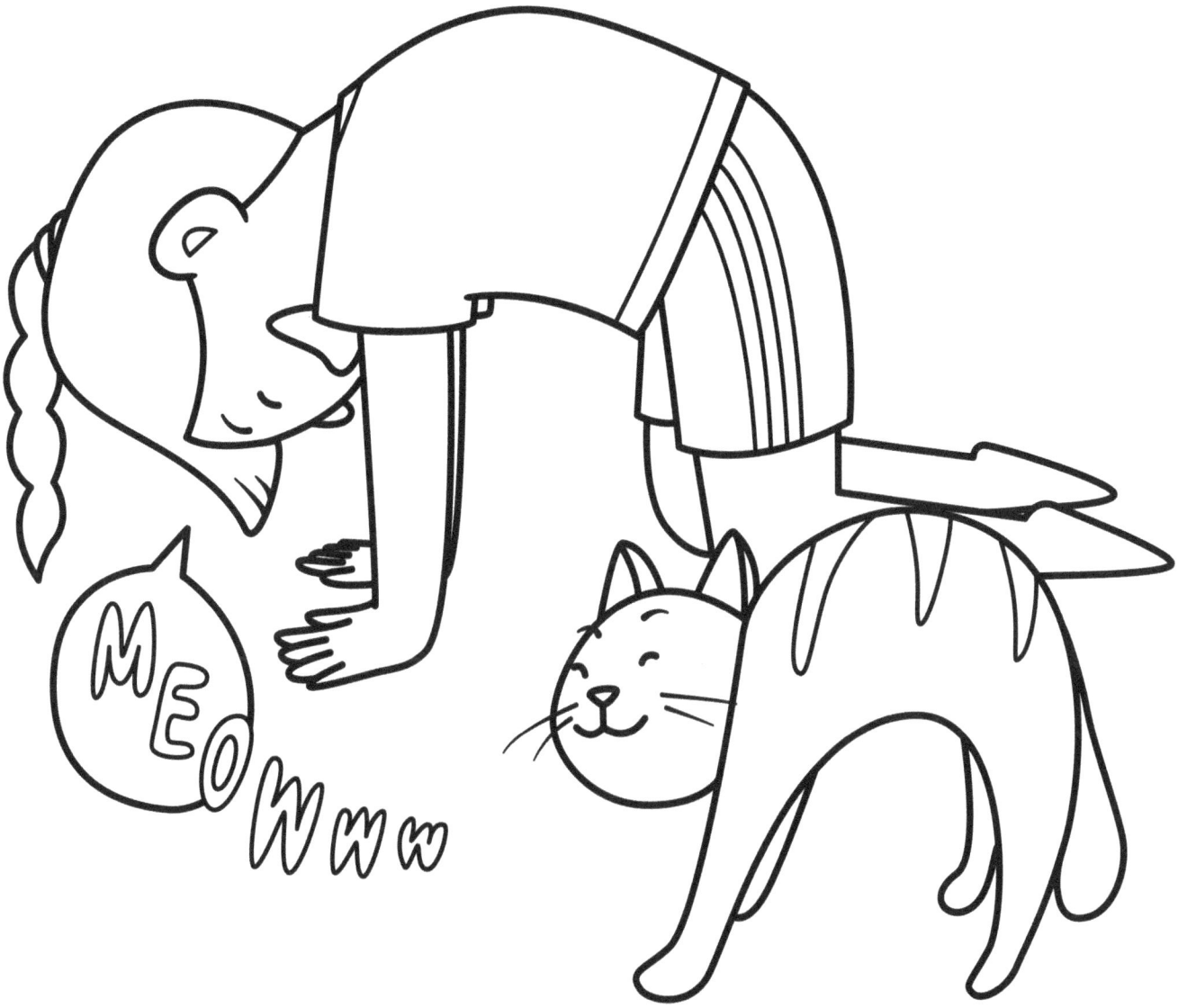

DOWNWARD DOG POSE

Great job, Happy Feet 'Little' Yogis! Ready to try a new pose that
will make us even stronger? Let's do the Downward Dog Pose!

From your "on all fours" position, with palms and knees on the mat,
keep your back straight. Lift your knees off the mat and raise your hips
towards the sky, forming a triangle shape with your body. Your head will be
between your arms, and your heels will reach towards the floor.
Feel the stretch in your spine and the strength in your back and legs.
Notice how this pose helps to calm your mind.

Can you give a big **WOOF WOOF**
like a playful and happy dog? Let's hear it!

Imagine someone crawling through the tunnel you've made with your body.
Hold your pose strong and steady —you're as strong as a superhero!

Let's say something awesome together:

"I AM STRONG!"

Feel the power in your body grow, like a superhero. It shines right through.
Hold your Downward Dog Pose for as long as it feels good.
You're doing amazing!

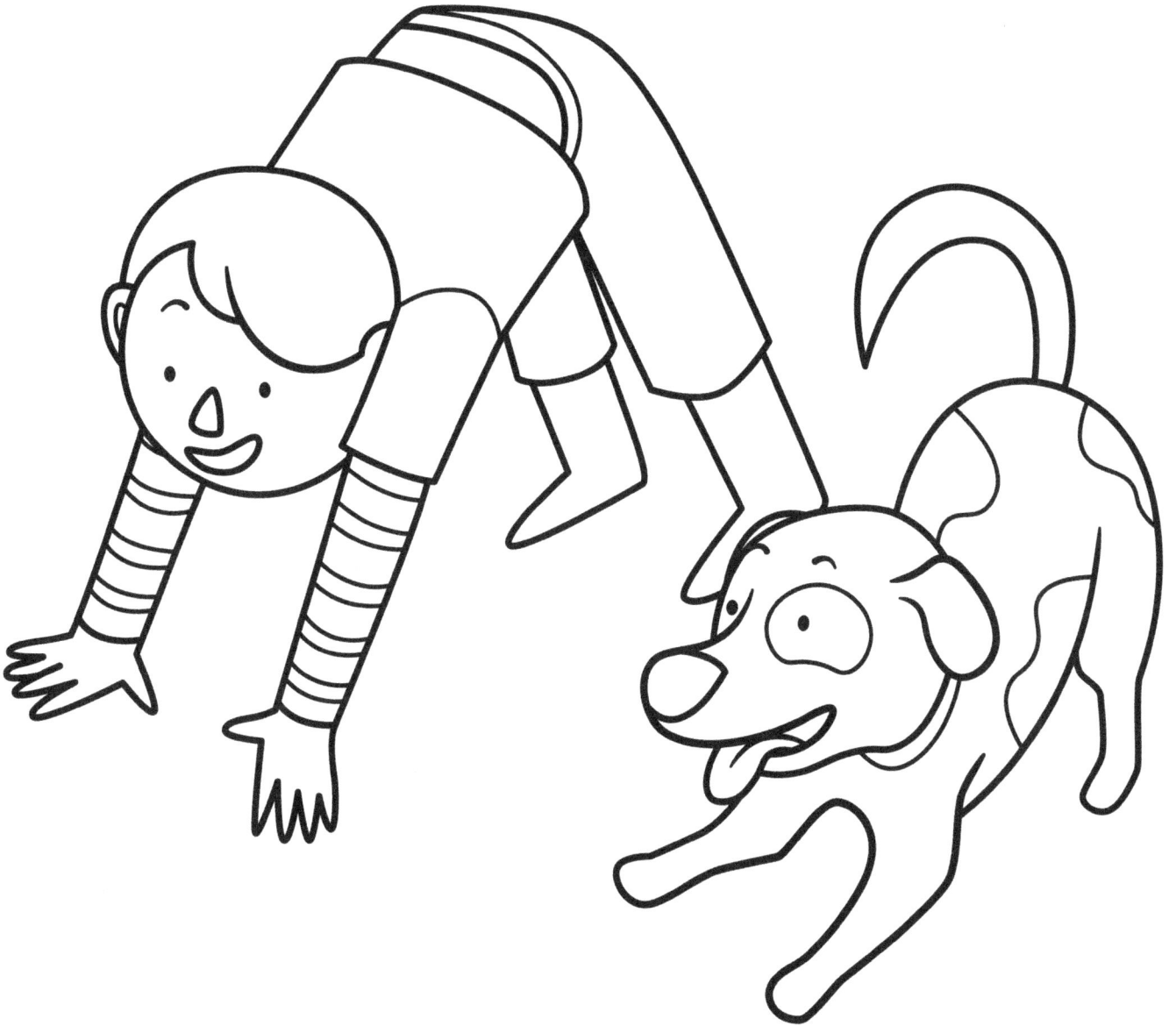

FROG POSE

Yay, Happy Feet 'Little' Yogis! Ready to ribbit like a frog
and jump high with the Frog Pose?

Sit on your mat or the floor. Bring your feet together, toes pointing
outwards, and spread your knees apart as much as you can.
Keep your back straight and find your balance.

Take a deep breath in through your nose. As you exhale, make a big
RIBBIT sound like a frog! Feel free to jump up high and land back in
Frog Pose. You can stay in one spot or hop around the room.

If you're feeling adventurous, have a froggy race! This pose opens your hips,
increases flexibility, and even helps with digestion. How cool is that?

If you are having fun, let's hear:

"I AM FUN!"

Feel the joy and excitement bubbling inside you like a playful frog.

Keep ribbiting, jumping, and having a blast, Happy Feet 'Little' Yogis!
You're spreading happiness and fun. Let's continue our yoga journey
with big smiles and lots of energy!

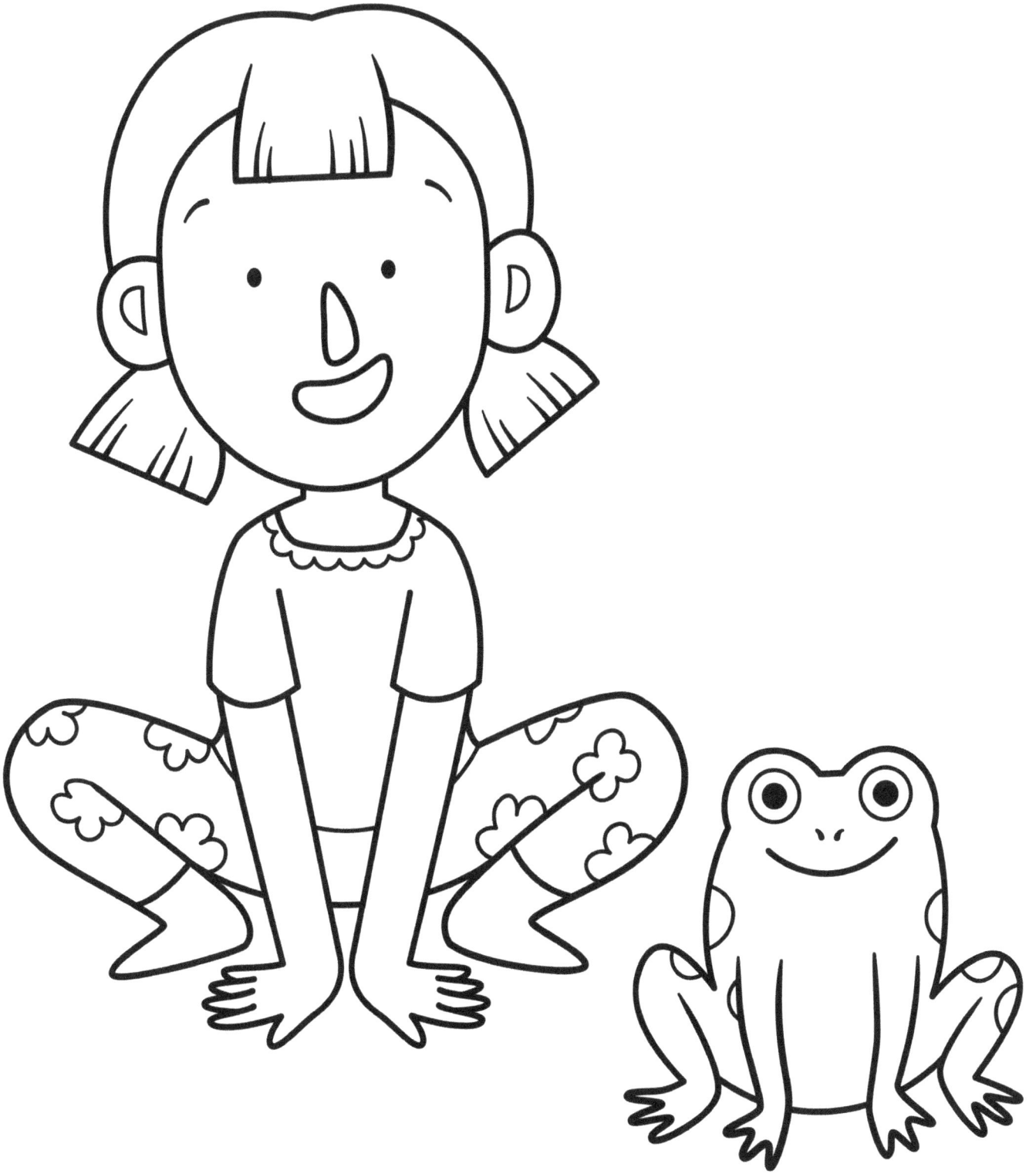

BUTTERFLY POSE

How wonderful, Happy Feet 'Little' Yogis!
Ready to transform into colourful butterflies?

Sit comfortably on your mat or the floor. Bring the soles of your feet together, letting your knees fall apart to open your hips. Keep your back straight and gently hold your feet with your hands.

Now, flap your wings like a butterfly! Touch your knees to the ground, then bring them back up. What colour is your butterfly today? Bright blue, sunny yellow, or a mix of all your favourite colours? Your butterfly can change colours every time we do this pose!

This Butterfly Pose helps open your hips and stretch your legs. It also makes your back and belly strong, and gives your body more energy and space to feel good.

Now, gently close your butterfly by bringing your chest towards the ground or your toes. Take a moment to relax and breathe deeply.

Let's feel the joy and say together:

"I AM LOVE!"

Feel the love and warmth spreading through you,
just like a butterfly spreading its wings.

Enjoy the peaceful feeling after our Butterfly Pose.
You're doing wonderfully! Let's continue our yoga journey with love and joy!

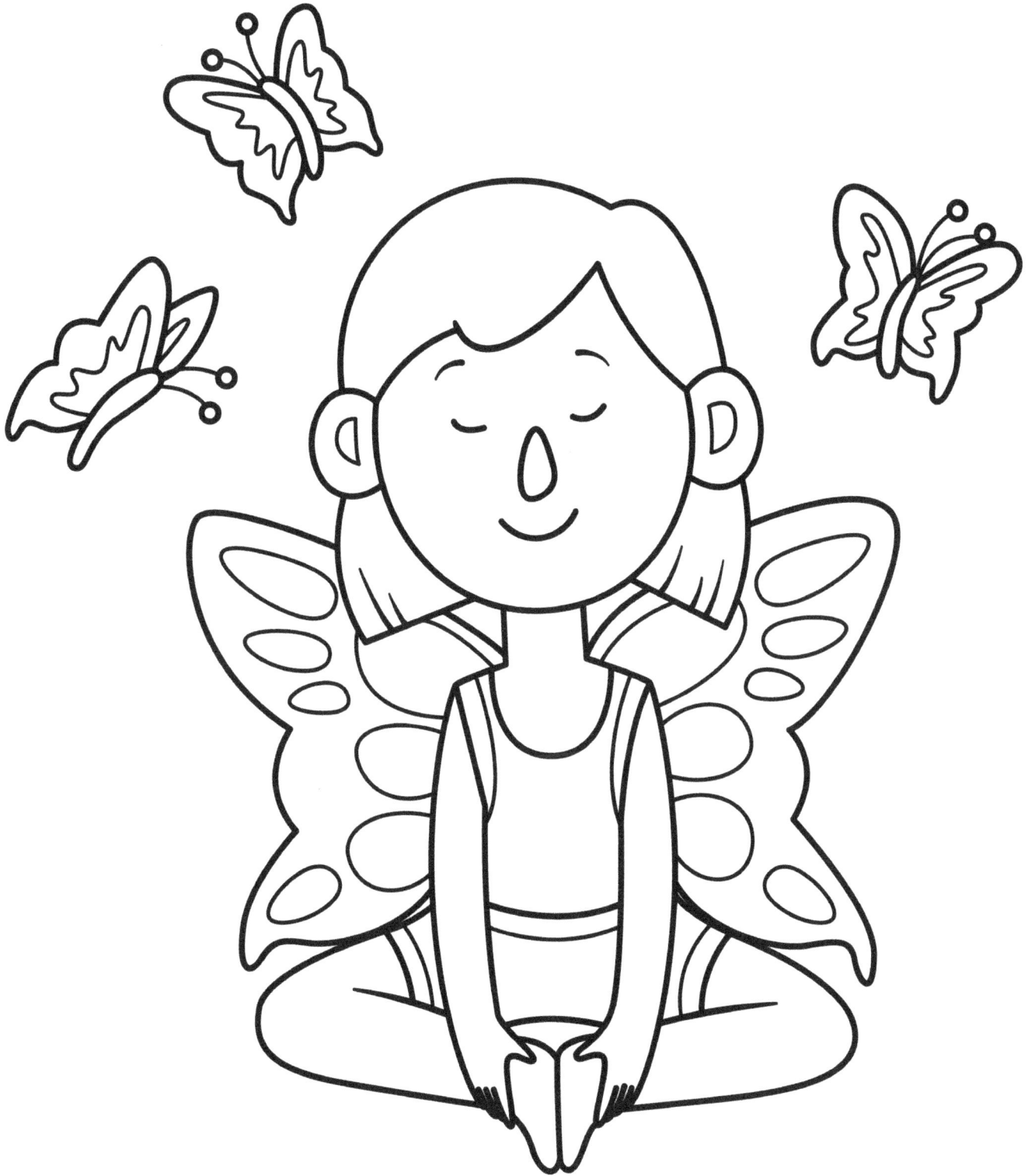

PEACOCK POSE

Great job, Happy Feet 'Little' Yogis! Ready to try our very own Peacock Pose? Sit comfortably on your mat with your legs in a V shape, keeping your knees straight. Gently reach towards your toes without bending your knees.

Can you feel the stretch in your back, legs, and hips?

In this pose, you stretch your back, and sit up tall like a mountain. It helps you stand and walk better too – that's called good posture! The more you breathe and stay in the pose, the more your blood moves all around your body, like a little river. Your legs and hips also get a nice stretch, so they feel more open and free to move.

Like a beautiful and colourful peacock, let's say:

"I AM CONFIDENT"

Feel the confidence and strength within you.

Enjoy the stretch and the sensation of being strong and flexible.
You're doing brilliantly! Keep practising and spreading beauty and positivity.
Let's continue our yoga adventure together!

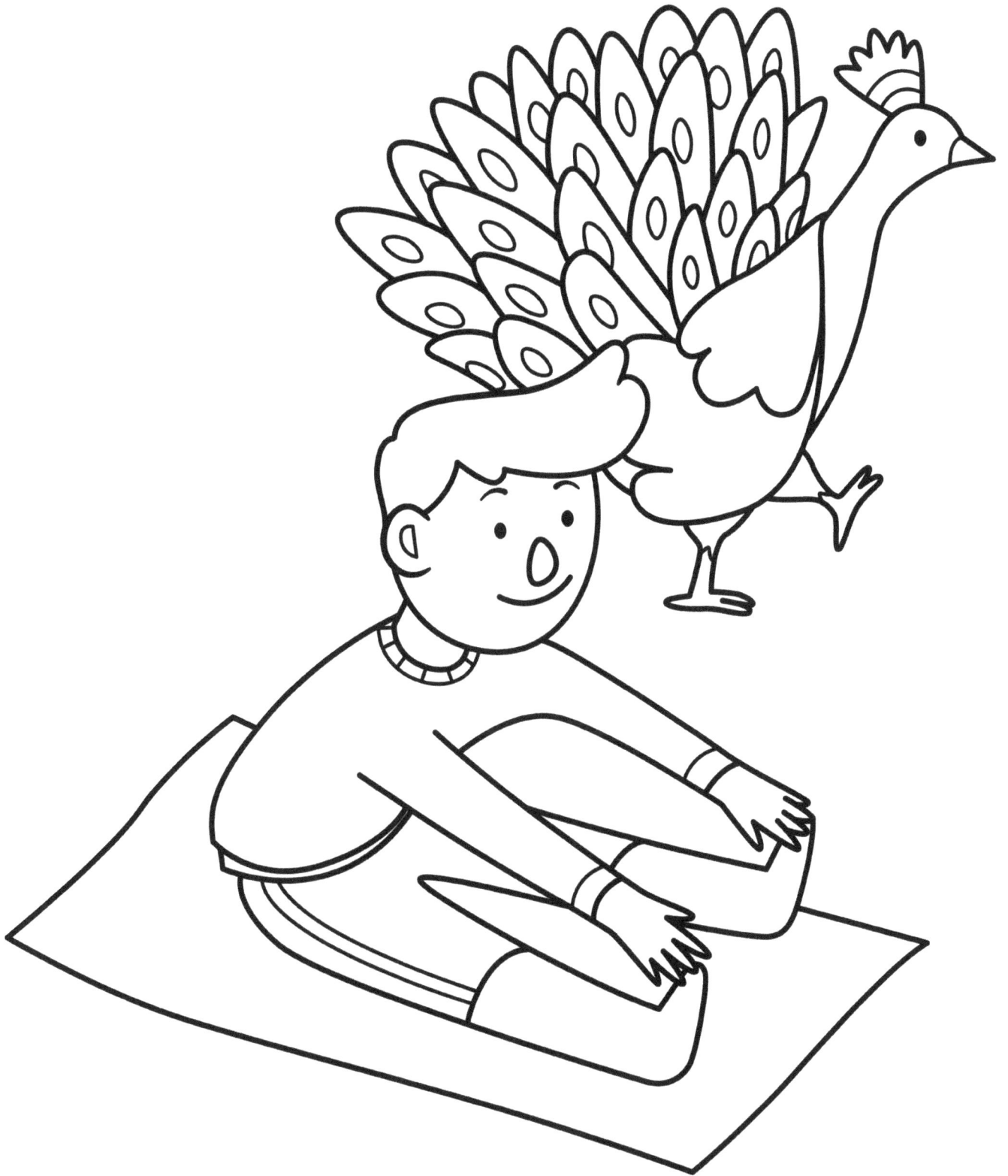

LOTUS POSE

Wow, Happy Feet 'Little' Yogis, let's transform into beautiful lotus flowers!
Ready for this challenge? You are brave and strong!

Sit comfortably with your legs stretched out in front of you.
Lift one leg and place the foot on the thigh of the other leg,
bending the knee gently. If this feels tricky, start with one side.
Hold for a few breaths, then switch sides.

If you're in the full Lotus Pose with both legs crossed, fantastic! Hold for a
few breaths. This pose opens up your hips and gives a nice stretch to your
ankles and knees. When you sit still and breathe here, it helps your body feel
calm and full of fresh energy – like you are recharging from inside.

For an extra challenge, place your hands next to your
hips on the mat, palms down. Lift your hips slightly and imagine
you're flying like a graceful lotus.

Can you feel it?

Like a beautiful and colourful lotus, let's say:

"I AM BEAUTIFUL!"

Feel the beauty and strength within you, like a lotus blooming in the sun.

Remember, yoga takes practice. You've come so far, and I'm impressed
with your determination! Keep practising and enjoying our yoga journey.
You're doing brilliantly!

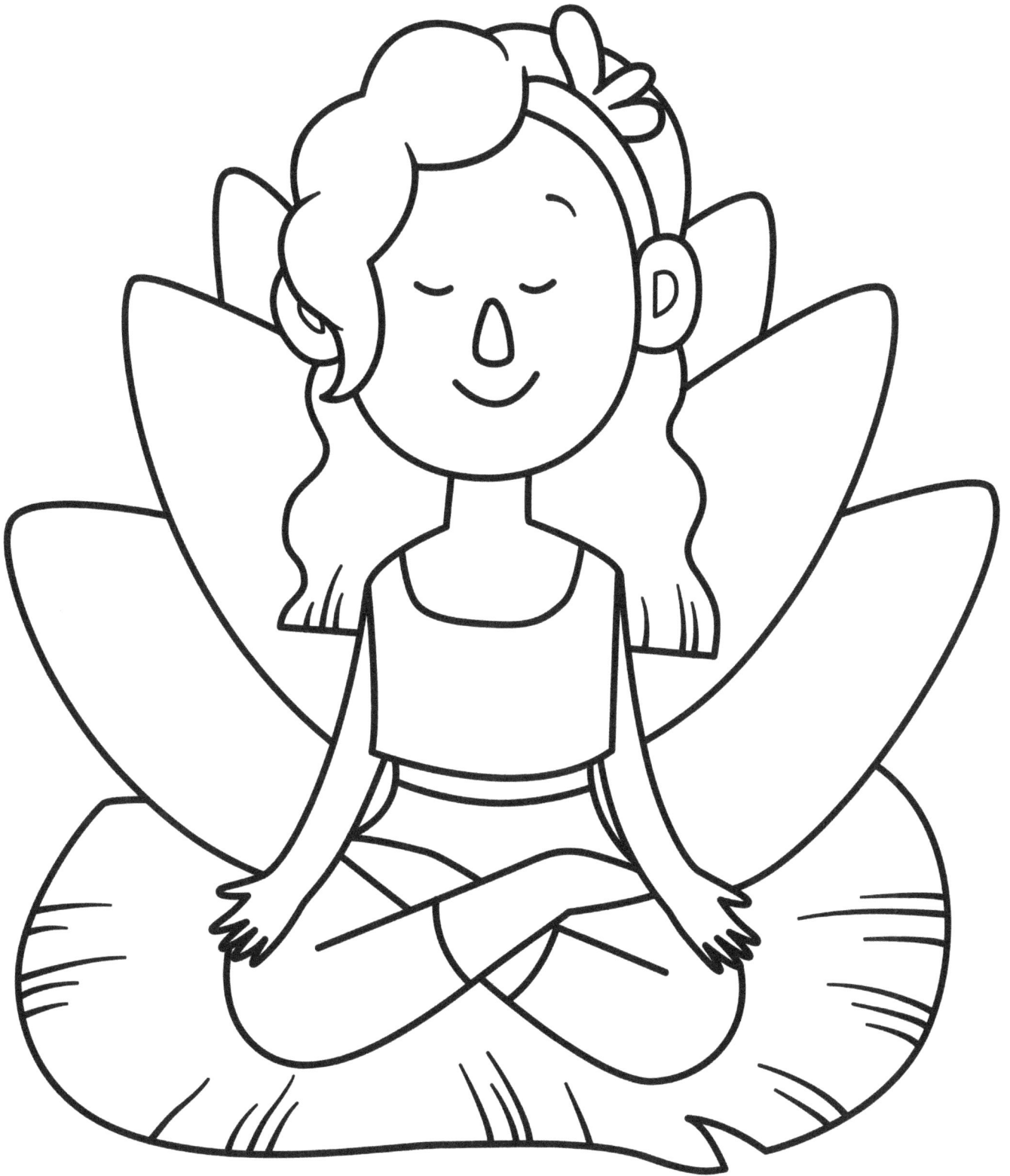

TREE POSE

It's time to stand tall, Happy Feet 'Little' Yogis! Let's try the
Tree Pose to become strong and balanced like a tree.

Stand on your feet. If you'd like, ask a loved one to support you
or practise together as a family! Imagine your foot is the tree root,
grounding you firmly. Lift your head and body high,
like the branches reaching towards the sky.

In the Tree Pose, balance on one leg and gently lift the other leg.
You can keep your hands at your sides, bring them together in
Namaste at your chest, or hold hands with your partner.

Focus on a fixed point, like a tree standing strong in the breeze.
The challenge is to be still and steady.

How do you feel in this pose? Say with me:

"I AM BRAVE"

Feel the courage and strength flowing through you,
like a mighty tree standing tall.

Take a deep breath and find your balance, like the tree standing strong in
the wind. Feel how your body becomes strong and steady like the branches
reaching to the sky with regular practice.

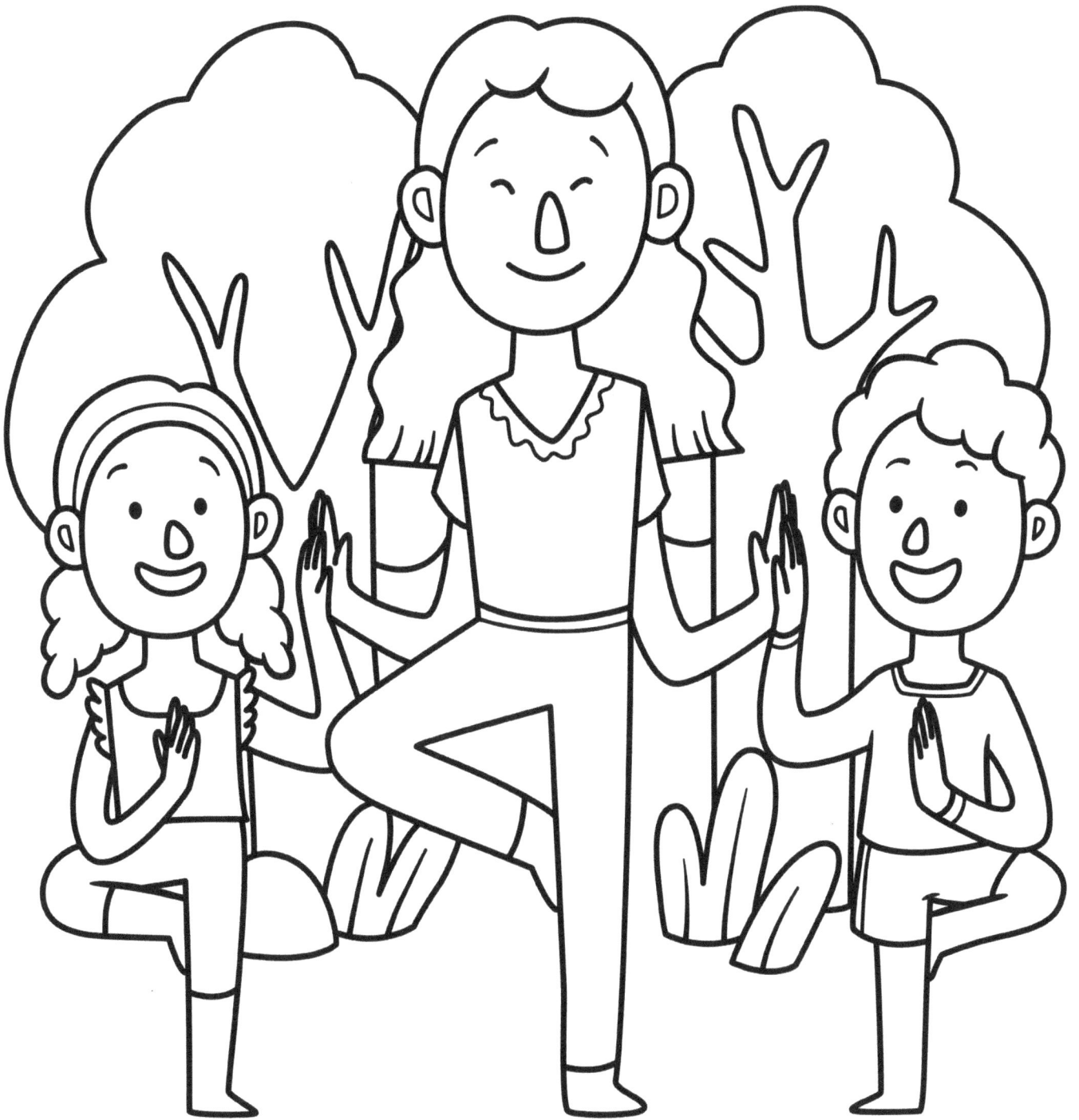

AIRPLANE POSE

Life is all about balance, Happy Feet 'Little' Yogis!
Ready for a fun balancing pose?
Imagine you're a plane flying through the air!

Stand tall on one leg, keeping both knees straight and strong.
Lift your other leg back as high as you can. Lean your upper body forward
to balance, and extend your arms out like airplane wings.
Look straight ahead, like a pilot focusing on the journey.

This pose helps make your back stronger and keeps you balanced like a
steady plane in the sky with more focus and confidence.

Try it on both legs, one side at a time!
Take your time and enjoy the feeling of flying.

Let's say something joyful together:

"I AM PLAYFUL!"

Feel the joy and playfulness spreading through you
like a plane soaring through the sky.

Keep practising and having fun, Happy Feet 'Little' Yogis!
You're doing amazing. Let's continue our yoga journey
with smiles and excitement!

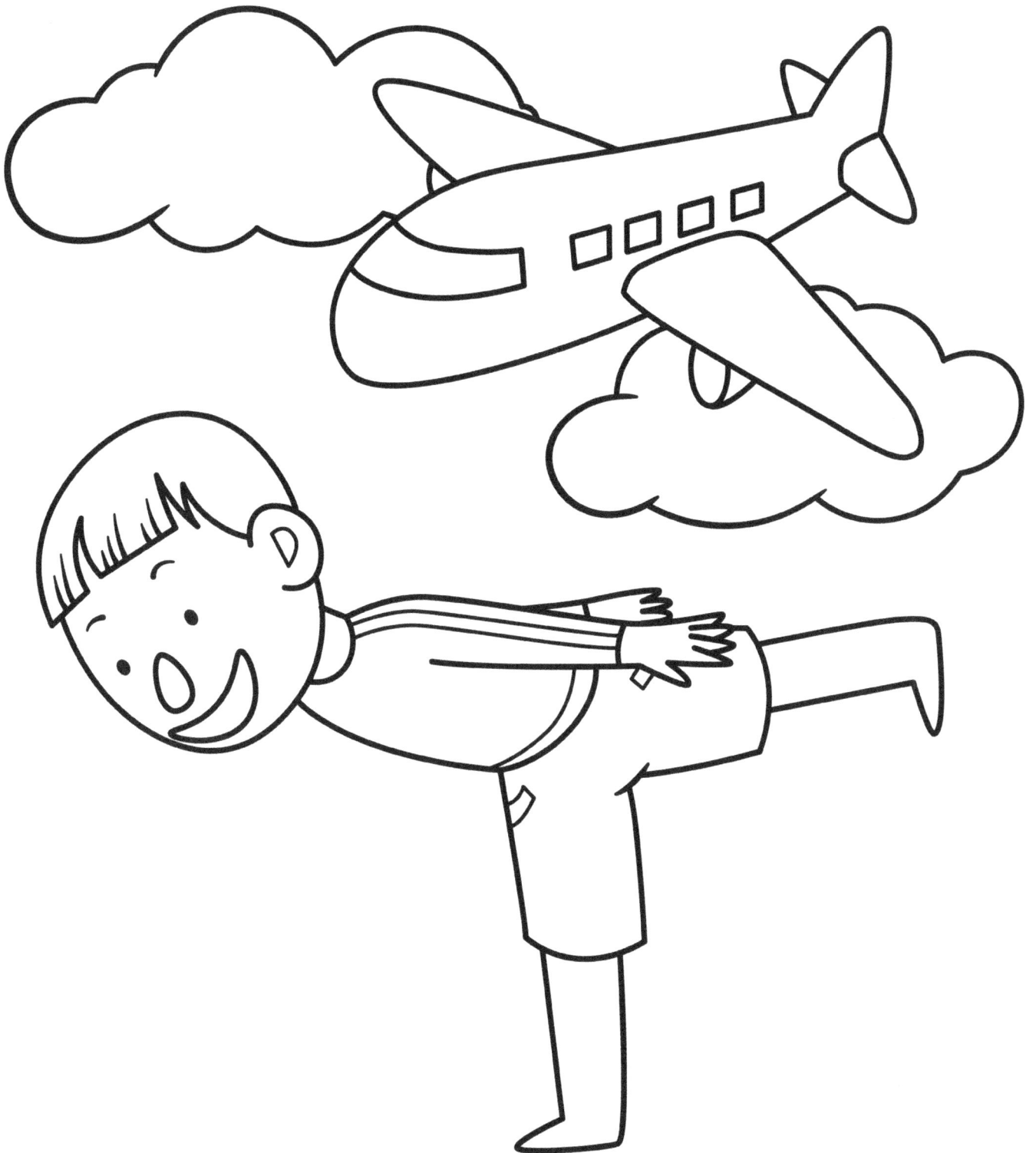

CANDLE POSE

Time to lie down on your back and light your candle,
Happy Feet 'Little' Yogis! Ready for a pose that will bring
strength and energy?

Lie on your mat and lift your legs and back off the ground,
pointing them straight up towards the sky. Keep your legs together
and your knees straight. Ask for help if needed to lift your back.

In the Candle Pose, imagine your toes are the candle's flame.
Hold this position like a bright, burning candle.

This pose makes your shoulders and back strong, like a superhero! It also
helps the blood flow in a new direction, which makes your whole body feel
fresh and happy.

Hold for a few seconds. When you're ready, make a wish
and blow out the candle with a big exhale.
Slowly lower your legs and back down, then relax.

Let's say something wonderful together:

"I AM BRIGHT!"

Feel the positivity filling you up like a shining candle.

Enjoy the relaxation after the Candle Pose. You're doing fantastic!
Keep shining brightly on our yoga journey together.

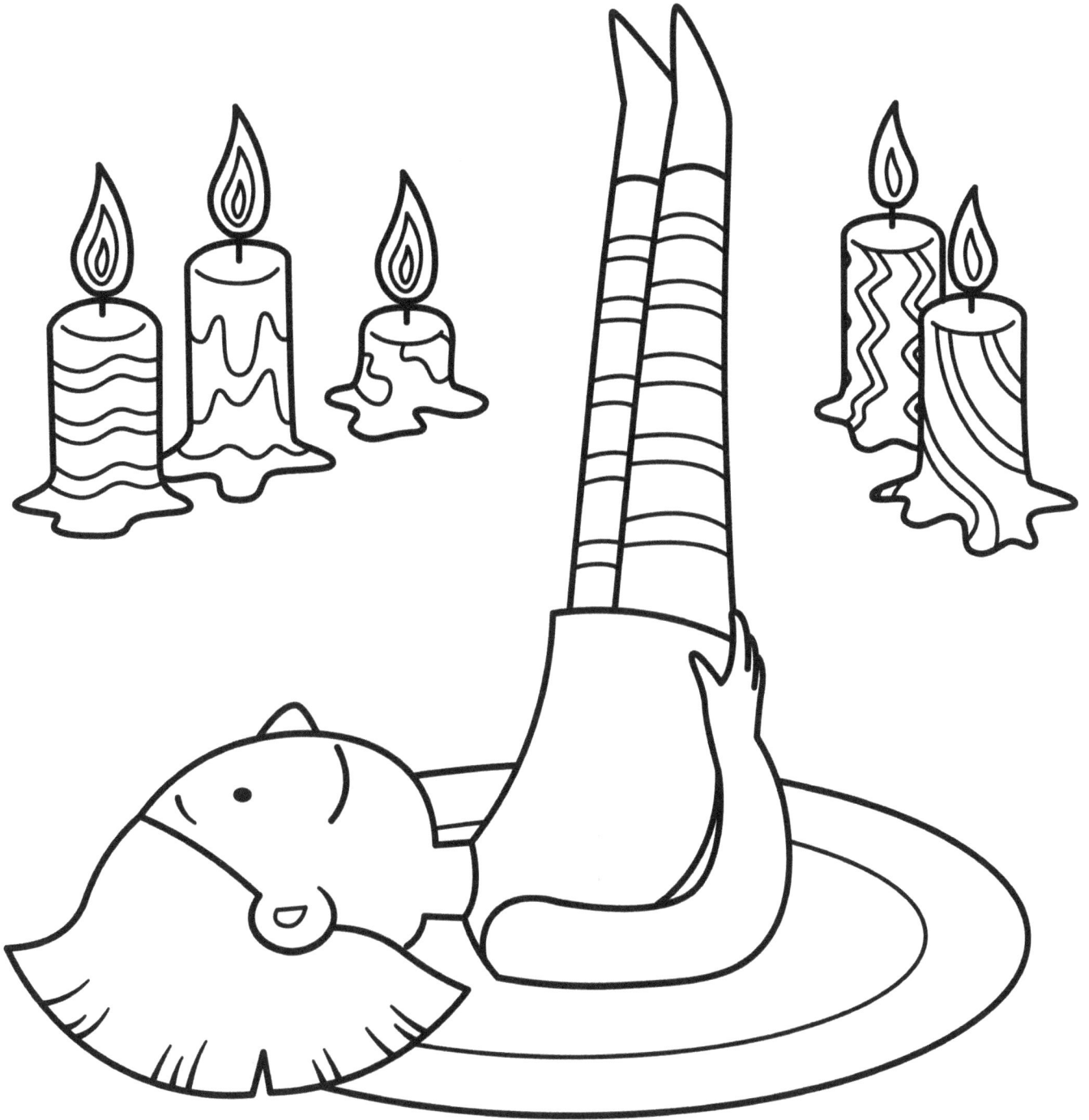

BRIDGE POSE

Let's keep making your back strong with the Bridge pose, Happy Feet 'Little' Yogis! Ready for this pose?

If you're still on your back from the Candle Pose,
bend your knees and bring your feet close to your hips,
leaving a small gap between your feet and knees.
If not, lie down on your mat.

Slowly lift your hips off the mat to create a bridge
with your back and strong legs. Feel the stretch in your
spine and the strength in your feet and legs.

Close your eyes for a few breaths and feel
the calmness spreading through you.

Let's say something wonderful together:

"I AM GRATEFUL!"

Feel the gratitude filling your heart, just like the
strength and stability you're building in the Bridge Pose.

Enjoy the relaxation and strength in the Bridge Pose,
Happy Feet 'Little' Yogis. You're doing brilliantly!
Keep up the great work on our yoga journey together!

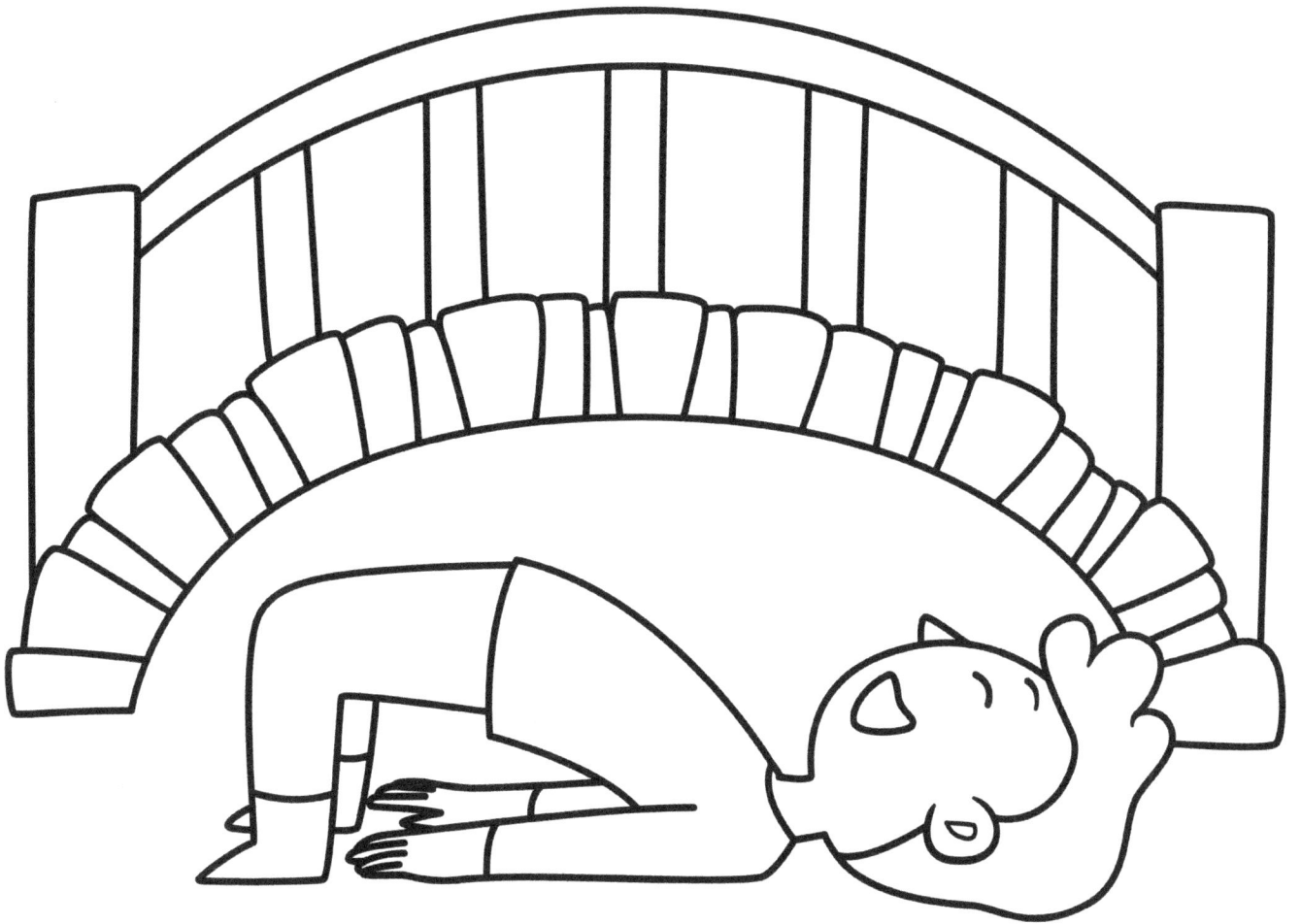

WHEEL POSE

Wow, Happy Feet 'Little' Yogis, let's finish our session strongly
with the Wheel Pose! Ready for this exciting challenge?
You've come so far, and you're going to love this pose!

Lie on your back on your mat. If you're coming from the Bridge Pose,
excellent! Place your hands close to your ears, with your fingers
pointing towards your shoulders.

Push through your hands and feet to lift into the Wheel Pose, creating an
arch with your spine. Feel the stretch in your upper body and the strength
in your arms and legs. This pose is a wonderful heart-opener!

If you need assistance, ask someone to gently support your lower back
as they help lift you up. Enjoy the openness and stretch as you rise.

Remember, the Wheel Pose can be challenging,
so take your time and hold the pose for a few breaths.

Let's speak some magic words from our heart:

"I AM FULL OF IMAGINATION!"

Feel the excitement and creativity moving through you, just like the strength
and stretch you feel in the chest and back with this pose.

Enjoy the happiness of the Wheel Pose, Happy Feet 'Little' Yogis.
You're doing brilliantly! Keep exploring and stretching your imagination
on our yoga journey together.

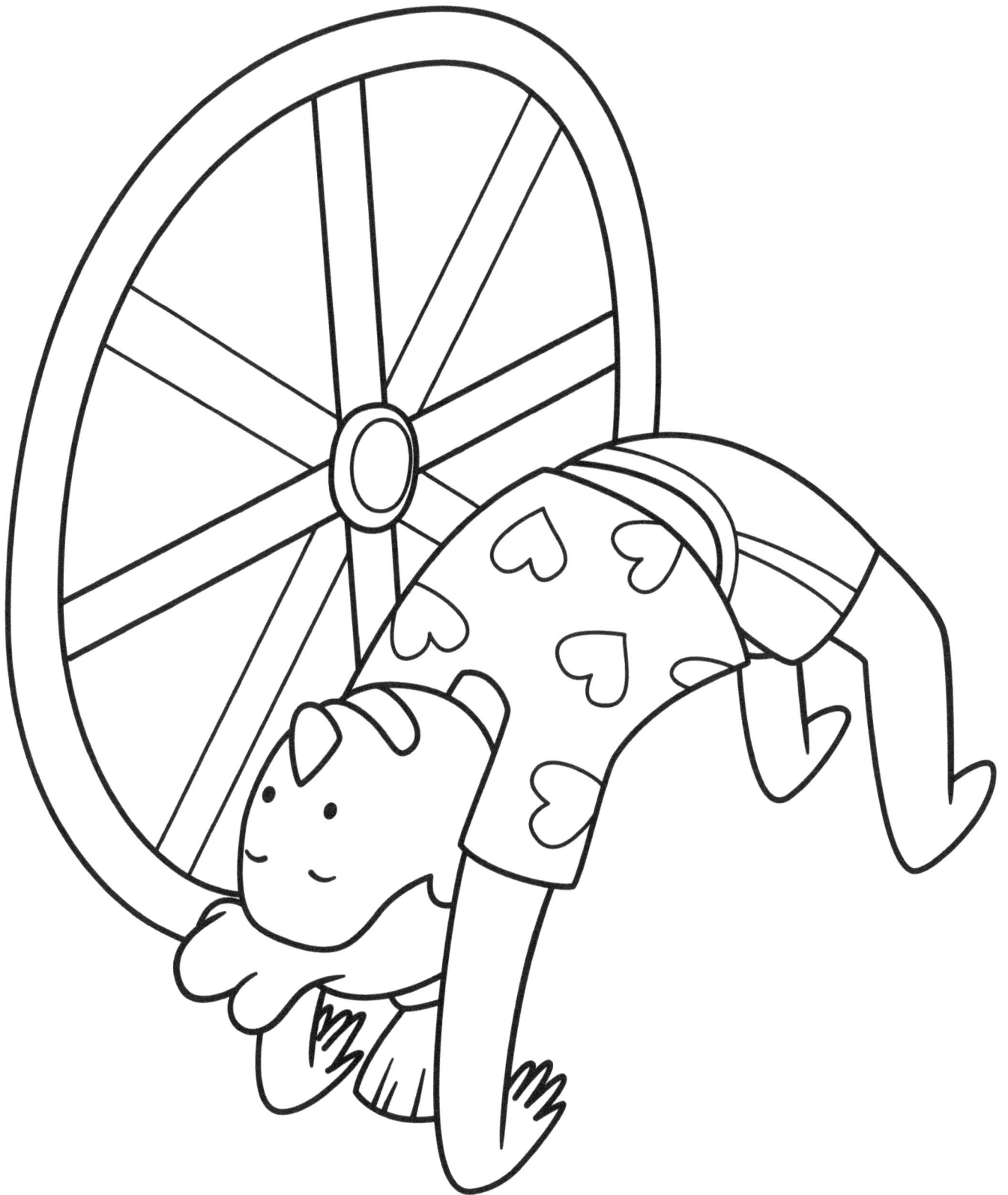

TO FINISH OUR FUN TIME, HAPPY FEET 'LITTLE' YOGIS, LET'S BRING EVERYTHING TOGETHER WITH A CALM AND THANKFUL MOMENT.

Are you ready?

First, bend your knees and give yourself a tight hug,
wrapping your arms around your legs. Thank your body
for this wonderful practice and all the strength and
flexibility it has shown.

Lie down on your back and remain in stillness,
as if peacefully sleeping. Take a few deep breaths here,
allowing your body to relax and absorb all the
benefits of your practice.

When you're ready, slowly come up to a seated position.
Let's finish our session just as we started, in Yogi Breath.
Sit comfortably with your legs crossed and bring your hands
together in prayer position at your heart.

Take a deep breath in, and as you breathe out,
let's say together:

NAMASTE!

Namaste means "the light in me honours the light in you".
It's a beautiful way to show respect and gratitude to each other
and to ourselves for the practice we've shared.

YOU DID AN AMAZING JOB, HAPPY FEET 'LITTLE' YOGIS! I'M SO PROUD OF YOUR FOCUS, STRENGTH, AND JOY THROUGHOUT OUR YOGA JOURNEY TOGETHER. KEEP PRACTISING AND SHINING BRIGHTLY. NAMASTE!

DEAR HAPPY FEET 'LITTLE' YOGI.

WELCOME TO YOUR SPECIAL JOURNAL WHERE YOU CAN CELEBRATE ALL THE WONDERFUL THINGS IN YOUR YOGA JOURNEY. LET'S BEGIN BY THINKING ABOUT WHAT FILLS YOUR HEART WITH HAPPINESS!

I AM THANKFUL!
TODAY I AM GRATEFUL FOR...

Write something that made you smile during our yoga time. Maybe it was a wiggly pose, a big belly breath, or just sharing a laugh with someone you love. Smiles are little treasures!

_____

_____

_____

_____

_____

_____

_____

I BELIEVE IN MYSELF!
MY SUPERPOWER BADGE IS...

Design your own badge that shows how amazing you are! It could be a symbol, an animal, or something totally made up. Maybe a tree for strong roots with tall and mighty branches, a butterfly for growth, or a star to shine bright!

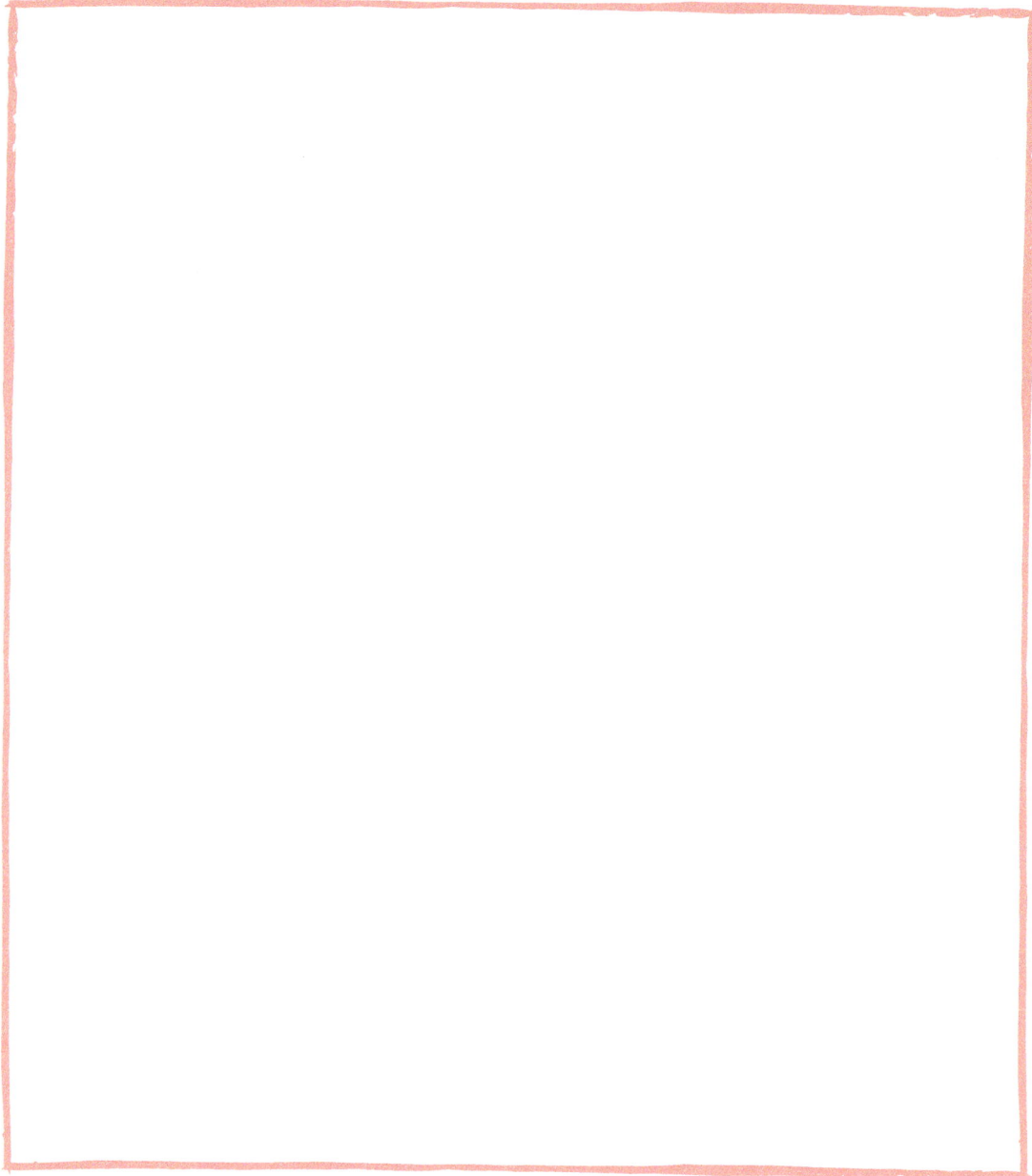

MY HEART IS FULL OF KINDNESS!
KINDNESS IS MAGIC, SO...

Write something kind you did today or something someone did for you. Maybe you helped a friend, shared your mat, or gave someone a compliment. Kindness is like sunshine—it warms everyone up!

_____

_____

_____

_____

_____

_____

_____

_____

MY BODY IS AMAZING!
TO CELEBRATE YOUR BODY...

Draw an outline of your body and fill it with anything you want. Be it colours, shapes, or stars. Your body helps you stretch, breathe, and play—it's truly magical!

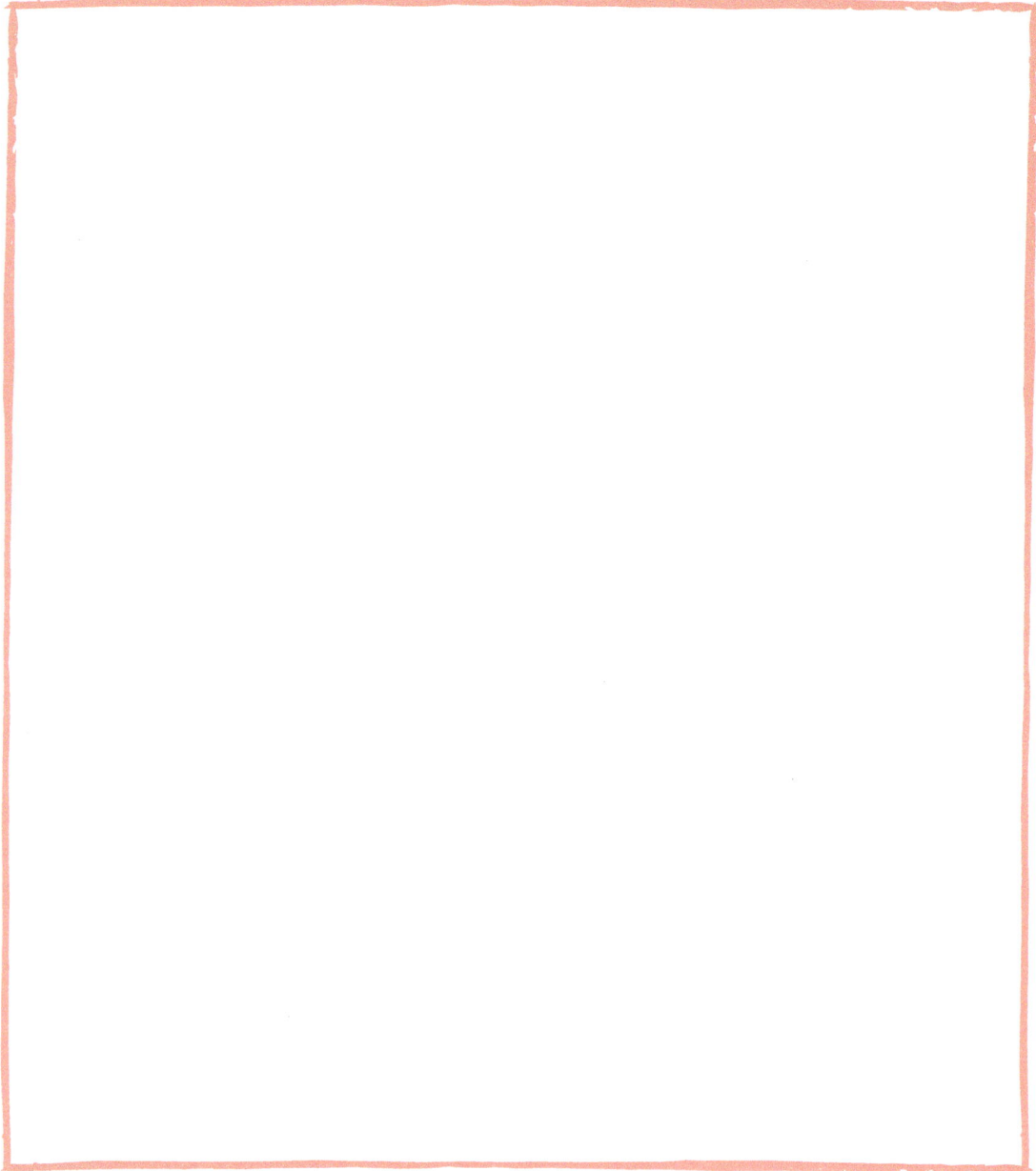

REMEMBER,

TAKE A MOMENT TO
BREATHE DEEPLY, FEELING THANKFUL
FOR ALL THE GOOD THINGS AROUND YOU.
BE KIND TO YOURSELF AND OTHERS, JUST
LIKE WE LEARN ON OUR YOGA MAT.

YOU ARE AMAZING AND UNIQUE,
SHINING BRIGHTLY IN OUR YOGA FAMILY!

MUCH LOVE AND NAMASTE!

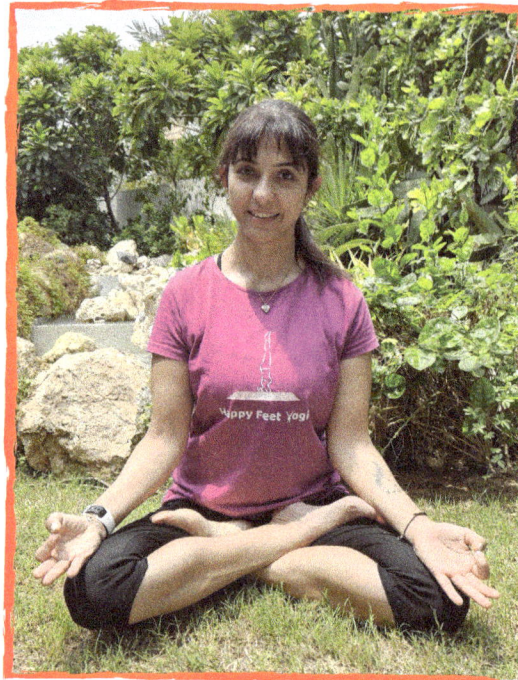

MEET BRINDA HORA, THE HEART AND SOUL BEHIND HAPPY FEET YOGI.

Hello, I'm Brinda Hora, the founder of Happy Feet Yogi.
My journey into yoga began in 2016, sparked by a transformative
personal experience that ignited a passion within me.
Since then, yoga has not only shaped my life but has also
inspired me to forge new paths with dedication and joy.

In 2020, I seized the opportunity to deepen my knowledge by pursuing Kids and Teens Yoga training. This experience resonated deeply with me, aligning perfectly with my vision for Happy Feet Yogi. Since then, I have had the privilege of connecting with children of all ages, starting at 3 years and upwards, guiding them through yoga sessions in private settings, small groups, and even camps with up to 25 kids per session.

I AM DEEPLY PASSIONATE ABOUT THE PROFOUND IMPACT YOGA CAN HAVE ON CHILDREN'S LIVES. IT FOSTERS SELF-DISCOVERY, INSTILS CALMNESS, AND NURTURES A GROUNDED SENSE OF RESPECT FOR OTHERS AND APPRECIATION FOR LIFE'S LITTLE JOYS.

Through yoga, children learn to work confidently on their own, alongside siblings, parents, or peers, thereby enhancing their social skills. Yoga also contributes to developing motor skills and coordination, complementing activities such as sports, gymnastics, and dancing. Furthermore, it cultivates concentration and mindfulness, which can significantly benefit academic performance and overall learning.

My dream is for yoga to become a natural part of every child's lifestyle, promoting awareness, mindfulness, and a deeper connection with their own body, mind, and breath. I envision a future where children embrace yoga not just as an activity, but as a holistic way of living that enriches their lives for years to come.

CONNECT WITH US:

happyfeetyogi.com

@happyfeet_yogi

@happyfeetyogi

@happyfeet_yogi